Raw Food

A BEGINNER'S GUIDE

Raw Food

A BEGINNER'S GUIDE

by
Anthea Wheal

GREEN

MAGIC

Green Magic
5 Stathe Cottages
Stathe
Somerset
TA7 0JL
England

www.greenmagicpublishing.com
email: info@greenmagicpublishing.com

Typeset by Green Man Books, Dorchester
www.greenmanbooks.co.uk

ISBN 978 0 9561886 6 3

GREEN MAGIC

CONTENTS

Introduction

v

To all of you who want to improve your lives.

INTRODUCTION

A diet consisting completely of raw food is unrealistic for the majority of us, but increasing your intake is a step in the right direction. Some is better than none.

Eating raw food is easy and just requires you to make a decision to give it a proper place in your diet. You do not have to eat only raw food straightaway – introduce your new diet slowly and as it feels good. If you rush it you may regret it.

The trick is to start off with your ordinary diet and then every now and then slip something raw in. Surprise yourself. It's nice to think that once you decide to go to raw or at least more raw you just do it and suddenly you are there. Experience teaches us that this is not how it works. You will find your digestion is not ready for it, and you may be kept awake for hours with a sore stomach wishing you had not rushed it. Your whole system needs adjusting to the new diet.

The 'five a day' portions of fruit and vegetables suggested by many experts is a great start to eating more raw food but we want to make this decision almost effortless, so you don't find yourself struggling on apple number five by the end of the day. The real key is making the recipes you try out tasty so that your meal doesn't become a chore to make and eat.

Some of the foodstuffs mentioned will not be items you would normally buy, but it's all about trying out new ideas and seeing what you can manageably incorporate into your everyday life. Quick, simple, nutritional and tasty dishes are what you are after to start with.

You will also find raw food an economical diet and that buying fresh food most days is an extremely positive way to approach life.

There are numerous health benefits from eating raw, or a high percentage of, raw food. From the recipes and ideas in this book, and from the way you will start to feel when increasing your raw food and decreasing your processed and cooked food intake, you will be able to judge how you are progressing and tune your diet to suit.

A true raw food diet consists only of foods which have not been heated above a certain temperature. The maximum temperature varies among the different forms of the diet, from 92°F to 118°F (33°C to 48°C)

Raw food diets may include raw fruits, raw vegetables raw nuts, raw seeds, raw unpasteurized dairy products (eg. milk, cream, butter), raw meat, raw eggs, and raw honey.

A *raw foodist* is a person who consumes primarily raw food. Raw foodists typically believe that the greater the percentage of raw food in the diet, the greater the health benefits. They generally believe raw food prevents and heals many forms of sickness and many chronic diseases.

Freezing food is considered acceptable by most raw food eaters. Many preserve nuts and seeds in the freezer.

Strictly speaking, most alcoholic drinks are produced from raw fruit and do not involve heat — the fermentation process not raising the temperature of the mix. This is a personal interpretation and you may feel that it's fine or you may feel that it is cheating.

Dehydrators are not mentioned in this book but when you are ready check them out. There are plenty of websites related to raw food and also plenty of mail order items that can fill in the gaps in your knowledge and your larder.

Eggs, sushi, dried meats and raw meats are not included in this book although you may wish to include these in your diet.

Just make sure that what you eat is what you want to eat, and not what you think you ought to eat.

'Let food be your medicine, and medicine be your food.'

Hippocrates (*c.* 460-370BC)

1. BREAKFASTS

A good start to the day can mean a glass of water, mashed banana and rolled oats or a full meal. Most people vary their start to the day every few weeks as the seasons change or simply because they crave something different. Maybe you have been away on holiday, or visiting a friend and seen what else people have for breakfast and so feel inspired to do something different.

Some things can be prepared before, some at the time and some can include both — it depends how you feel first thing. It always used to be said that breakfast was the most important meal of the day so take it seriously. People who skip breakfast are more likely to have problems with concentration and their metabolism.

Smoothies make a great breakfast and also just eating fruit on its own can be perfect but let's assume you've looked at those options and want something different, so here are suggestions for a variety of easily made things to eat to get you going if you are hungry!

Apple and Avocado Purée

1 avocado
2 apples
¼ cup purified water

Peel the apples and take out the core. Take the avocado meat out of the skin and discard stone. Put the two ingredients in a bowl and blend with the water until smooth.

Buckwheat Breakfast

1 cup sprouted buckwheat
8 soaked dates
1 apple
2 tbsp shredded coconut
Fresh cinnamon to taste

Put everything in a blender or food processor for 30 seconds.

Muesli

6 apples
1 cup rolled oats
¼ cup raisins
½ tsp cinnamon

Juice the apples and, in a bowl, combine the apple juice and pulp with the oats, raisins, almonds and cinnamon.

Cover the bowl and place in the fridge to soak overnight.

Pour the muesli into a bowl and add slices of fresh fruit.

Breakfast Crunch

1 small sweet potato, peeled (grated or flaked)
¼ cup almonds or walnuts (chopped and
    soaked)
1 sliced banana
Sweet almond milk

Mix ingredients together and pour almond
milk on top.

Breakfast Mix

1 celery stalk
1 small apple
1 pear
1 kiwi fruit
1 tsp ground cinnamon
1 tbsp ground up flaxseeds

Peel and chop the fruits. Mix into the celery
in a bowl.
Sprinkle the cinnamon and flaxseeds on top.

Classic Breakfast Juice or Fruit

Apple
Cranberry
Grapefruit
Mango
Orange
Pineapple

Carrot Juice

2 lbs carrots
½ lemon

Wash the lemon and cut most of the peel off.
Juice the lemon and the carrots together.

Banana and Coconut Pancakes

1 banana
2 tbsp coconut meal or dried coconut flakes
Pinch ground cinnamon

Mash the banana with a fork in a bowl until very smooth. Mix in the coconut and cinnamon. Flatten into small pancakes.

Leave out in direct sunlight for about 1 hour, flip over and leave for another hour until dry to the touch.

Simple Porridge

3 cups rolled oats (soaked)
2 tbsp coconut butter
1 tbsp agave syrup
Pinch salt
1 cup water

Soak the oats for 20 minutes in water. Drain them, then add everything else and blend until smooth.

Fancy Porridge

6 fresh stoned dates
½ cup almonds
½ cup walnuts
½ cup oats
2 peeled and cored apples
¼ tsp vanilla extract
1 tsp lemon juice
¼ tsp ground cinnamon
⅛ tsp peeled and chopped ginger

Blend nuts, oats and dates. Then add the rest to the blender and give it another quick pulse.

2. SMOOTHIES AND JUICES

Smoothies and juices are the quickest and easiest way for busy people to consume a large amount of fruit and vegetables, as they fit in just one glass. Adding ice, crushed or cubed, improves the taste no end.

Once you have a feel for what you like it's easy to tailor the recipes to suit your mood, by either adding, subtracting or substituting ingredients. Drinks make a wonderful breakfast and are very invigorating. Do remember that a large cold drink on a frosty morning can make you feel cold too so do use your common sense.

There are plenty of ready-made products on shelves in all types of shops. But if you are making your own then you know exactly what the ingredients are, and you can control the amount and mixture to get just the sensation you need. It involves minimal washing up and the cost will be less too.

Here are some easy to make and delicious mixtures and ideas to base your own blends and styles around.

Minty Smoothie

2 medium bananas
1 medium cucumber
2 tbsp fresh basil
1 tbsp fresh mint
2 stoned peaches

Blend until smooth.

Oats and Banana

2 small bananas
8fl oz ice cold milk
1 tbsp rolled porridge oats
2 ice cubes

Blend until smooth.

Cinnamon Smoothie

2 bananas
1 small cup frozen rasberries
1 small cup frozen blueberries
1 small cup pure orange juice
1 tsp vanilla essence
1 tsp maple syrup
3 ice cubes
Cinnamon to taste

Blend until smooth.

Berries and Banana

¼ cup fresh or frozen assorted berries
1 small banana
1 cup pure orange juice
4 tbsp of low fat vanilla yoghurt

Blend until smooth.

Blackberries and Melon

2 cups frozen blackberries
2 cups honeydew melon (fresh or frozen)

Blend until smooth.

Pineapple and Bananas

2 large ripe bananas cut into spieces
4 tbsp low-fat natural yoghurt
9fl oz pineapple juice

Blend the bananas, pour in the pineapple juice followed by the yoghurt. Blend until smooth.

Fruitiferous

2 slices pineapple
1 tbsp pineapple juice
1 small cup red grapes
1 small cup white grapes
2 ice-cubes

Blend until smooth.

Fruity Cup

5 strawberries
1 banana
8 raspberries
1 clementine, peeled
3 ice cubes

First blend the fruits together, then add the ice.

Strawnana

2 large ripe bananas
8 strawberries
1 pear, peeled and cored
2 peeled kiwi fruits
14fl oz fresh blackcurrant juice

Blend all together until smooth.

Vegetable Smoothie

1   tbsp lemon juice
1   cup broccoli
1   chopped tomato
1   small chopped carrot,
1   cup kale
½ cup hulled sunflower seeds
1   peeled garlic clove
½ cup sesame seeds
2   slices peeled onion

Blend all ingredients till smooth.

Mark's Lemon and Mint Treat

Handful of fresh mint
Juice of 1½ lemons
1 tbsp agave nectar
4 cups of hot water
4 cups of ice cubes

Spoon the agave into the hot water and stir well then blend everything together till smooth.

Fruit Juices

There are many fruits that can be pressed cold to obtain the juice. We all know apple juice, orange and cranberry but there are a surprisingly large number of others and they are a useful addition to the raw diet as cups of hot tea and coffee are now off the menu. Then of course there are all the different mixes that can be tried out. ....

Persian Yoghurt Drink - Dugh

2½ cups plain whole-milk yoghurt
1 tbsp dried mint leaves —
   keep a pinch for decoration
1 tbsp dried rose petals —
   keep a pinch for decoration
Pinch salt
Pinch black pepper
2 pints cold water
A few ice cubes

Mix the yoghurt with the mint, rose petals, salt and pepper. Add the water and ice cubes, mix up and sprinkle with decoration.

Lassi

Lassi is traditional Indian drink based on yoghurt. It is made by blending yoghurt with water or milk and spices. Traditionally lassi is a drink that is savory and can have ground roasted cumin added for taste while the sweet style lassi can be blended with fruits or sweet ingredients.

Mango Lassi

7fl oz untreated milk
14fl oz natural unsweetened yoghurt
14fl oz mango pulp
4 tsp caster sugar

Blend the ingredients together and serve over ice.

Traditional Salty Lassi

4 cups yoghurt
3 cups cold water
1 cup crushed ice
2 small fresh chopped green chili peppers
1 tsp cumin, roasted and ground
3 tbsp lime or lemon juice
2 tsp salt

Combine all ingredients except ice in blender and blend until smooth. Then add ice and continue blending until frothy.

Kefir

Kefir is a cultured, enzyme-rich food with micro-organisms that help balance your diet. It is more nutritious than yoghurt, supplying protein, minerals and B vitamins. Kefir is simple and inexpensive to make at home and can also be used to restore the gut after antibiotic therapy. Kefir can be made into a delicious smoothie. To make perfect kefir you will need to use the internet for recipes and order up a small starter kit.

Time and temperature are the key factors that determine how your kefir will turn out. In the warmer months kefir may be ready to drink in under a day. If you let it sit out too long it will turn to cheese. If your kefir is lumpy, you are definitely leaving it out too long. It should be creamy and drinkable — a little thicker than milk. At this point, shake it well and place the kefir in the fridge. It will thicken a little more since it is continuing to culture, but more slowly. With eachbatch, change the time until it comes out just the way you like it.

After you start your first batch of kefir you can use a small amount of it to make your second batch. How much to use is included in the instructions found in each package of starter. If you transfer too much kefir from one batch to the next, you'll create a product that cultures too fast and tastes too sour. You can do this about 7 times from one batch to the next. After that, the yeast starts to get spoiled.

3. SOUPS

The oldest form of prepared food is said by many to be soup. Soup is great anytime of the year and involves much less chewing than just vegetables or salad. A very small bowl can be eaten whilst preparing something more substantial or even as a delicate little item on its own between meals to keep you going.

A spoonful of plain yoghurt makes a great add on to most soups as does sprinkling fresh and finely chopped or minced herbs on top just before serving.

We all think of hot soups in the winter as the traditional style but here are a few ideas that are not like that at all. It's all about good strong flavors. Although in cold weather cold soup may not be first on your list.

Soup is very digestible and nourishing and can be quickly made and eaten with a nice snack on the side too.

Gaspacho Soup

½ cup of each: corn, red pepper, and
  cucumber
¼ cup of each: zucchini and onion
2 tbsp parsley
1 tbsp cilantro
½ clove chopped peeled garlic
1 tbsp water or juice

Blend red pepper. Add cucumber and
corn, blend until smooth. Add remaining
ingredients, blend thoroughly, add water or
juice for consistency.

Celery, Onion and Carrot Soup

2 or 3 carrots
1 red onion
3 celery sticks
1 tsp coriander seed
Pinch black peppercorns
Pinch salt
1½ cups water

Wash, peel and trim as necessary. Chop the
carrots, onion and celery and place in blender.
Grind the coriander seed and peppercorns with
a pinch of salt and briefly blend, then add the
water and blend till smooth. Heat in a small
pan, stirring occasionally until just warm.

Cucumber Soup

1 peeled cucumber
½ peeled avocado
5 sprigs fresh chives
12 raw cashews, soaked in cold water for 12
    hours
1 small garlic clove peeled
Pinch salt and pepper
1 tbsp water

Blend everything, except half the avocado
and water, till smooth and if too thick add a
spoonful of water. Garnish with the rest of the
avocado sliced thinly, and eat straightaway.

Carrot and Avocado Soup

½ pint carrot juice
2 peeled avocados
½ tsp dulse flakes
½ oz fresh ginger
¼ tsp cayenne
1 small garlic clove
1 medium onion

Blend all together in blender or if you like it chunky just blend avocado, ginger, garlic, and juice together. Then add chopped onions, cayenne and broken up pieces of dulse flakes.

Melon Soup

2 cups chopped cantaloupe
2 cups chopped watermelon
2 cups fresh raspberries
2 cups chopped honeydew melon
1 cup chopped mango or banana
Juice of a lime
2 tbsp raw honey or raw agave nectar
cinnamon to taste

Put canteloupe and raspberries into bowls.

Blend everything else in blender until smooth and pour over fruit in bowls. Sprinkle with ground cinnamon.

Spinach Soup

3 small avocados
Handful of spinach
2 small lemons deseeded and chopped
2 red bell peppers
3 cups water
1 jalapeno pepper

Blend all together until smooth.

Mango and Tomato Soup

1 peeled and stoned chopped mango
6 cherry tomatoes
2 cups spinach
½ cup water

Blend the water, mango and tomatoes briefly then add the spinach and blend until smooth.

Pepper Soup

5 medium tomatoes
½ chopped cucumber
1 red bell pepper
2 cloves peeled and chopped garlic
¼ cup water
¼ tsp cayenne
2 tbsp fresh chopped parsley
1 chopped peeled avocado

Blend together all ingredients except parsley and avocado until smooth. Stir in the avocado and parsley. Put in fridge for three hours to let the flavors develop. Serve cold.

Fancy Butternut Squash Soup

3 cups butternut squash, peeled, seeded
   and chopped
1 mango, cubed
2 tsp curry powder
4 cups orange juice
½ cup honey or dates

For garnish:

1 plantain or banana, peeled and sliced
½ cup chopped fresh mint
Pinch minced jalapeno
1 mango, seeded, peeled and diced

In a blender, combine the butternut
squash, mango, curry powder, orange
juice, and honey or dates and blend until
creamy. Sprinkle with plantain or banana
slices, mint, jalapeno, and mango.

Classic Spinach Soup

Bunch of spinach leaves
½ cucumber, peeled
¼ cup water
1 peeled and stoned avocado
1 clove peeled garlic
2 tbsp organic soy sauce
Pinch salt
Pinch black pepper ground
Pinch chili powder
1 tbsp lemon juice
1 tbsp olive oil

Blend all ingredients till smooth.

Spicy Celery Soup

3 celery stalks
1 yellow bell pepper
5 tomatoes
2 small zuccini
1 tsp chili powder
1 tsp ground flax seeds
1 clove peeled garlic
4fl oz water

Add the water and tomatoes and blend briefly. Then add the rest and blend till smooth.

Tomato Soup

1 red pepper
4 large ripe tomatoes
5 tsp olive oil
1 tsp fresh ginger grated
4 small fresh onions
Pinch of cayenne
Pinch of salt
Pinch of cinnamon

Blend until smooth adding water if too thick.

4. MAIN MEALS

When you need food the best thing to do is to go out and get what you fancy there and then. When you get in it can just be put together and eaten at once — the best! However it's always true to say that not every day works out this way, so a bit of forethought and planning can be very handy too.

It is important to sit down and have a full meal once a day to both ground you and give you the strength and balance to get everything done. Raw food is very energising but also can be harder work to digest than cooked or processed foods, so do allow time for a meal to go down before you dash out the door again.

These recipes are really ideas for you to think about and expand upon, they are not fixed but something for you to hang your own ideas on. They are also perfectly good as they are.

Lunch Feast

1 peeled and sliced banana
1 chopped and cored apple
2 tbsp oats
2 tbsp raisins
2 tbsp pecans
1 tsp organic honey

Mix everything together and pour the honey on top.

Lunch Bowl

2 large chopped tomatoes
½ small red onion very finely chopped
2 crushed cloves of peeled garlic
½ jalapeno pepper finely minced
Juice of 1 lemon
½ cup chopped cilantro leaves
Large pinch salt
1 tbsp sun-dried tomato paste

Mix everything together and leave for 45
minutes.

Fabulous Zucchini Mix

16 oz cherry tomatoes
3 zucchini
½ small onion
6 basil leaves
2 peeled cloves garlic
1 red bell pepper
2 tsp mixed dried spices
Olive oil to suit

Shred the zucchini finely and put to one side. Blend all other ingredients to a rough consistency but not for too long. Pour the sauce into a bowl and allow to thicken for 30 minutes. Pour the sauce over the zucchini and serve.

Veggie Burger

1 large peeled and chopped onion
1 deseeded bell pepper
3 carrots
10 oz chopped cauliflower
6 oz chopped broccoli
1 cup almonds, soaked for 24 hours
1 cup sunflower seeds, soaked for 6 hours
¼ cup sesame seeds, soaked for 6 hours
4 cloves peeled garlic
¼ tsp cumin seeds
2 tsp soy sauce
2 tsp fresh cilantro leaves

Blend everything in a food processor. Mould into ½ inch thick burgers on a tray and place in fridge for 24 hours.

Chili Warmer

1 cup water
1 cup pre-soaked sun-dried tomatoes
½ cup olive oil
2 tbsp lemon juice
2 cloves peeled garlic
1 tsp chili powder
Pinch salt

Blend all ingredients. Then add and stir in:

2 cups chopped tomatoes
1 cup sliced mushrooms
1 cup chopped celery
Handful chopped basil

Sprinkle with chopped parsley.

Burrito

1 mashed avocado
1 diced yellow pepper
1 finely sliced red onion
3 seeded and chopped red jalapeno peppers

Mix them all together and spoon into whole red cabbage or lettuce leaves. Squeeze lime juice over the top and wrap each leaf.

Sandwich

2 romaine lettuce leaves
10 slices cucumber
1 sliced tomato
8 slices red onion

Slap everything on a leaf with a bit of your handiest or favorite dressing, adding the top leaf and eating at once.

Tomato Sandwich

1 thickly sliced very large ripe tomato
1 finely grated zucchini
1 finely grated squash
1 thinly sliced onion
1 mashed avocado
Pinch thyme or basil

On one slice of tomato, place the zucchini and squash and onion. Put avocado on top. Sprinkle on herbs. Place second slice of tomato on top.

Vital Rounds

1 cup walnuts or pecans
1 cup sprouted wheat berries
  (soak ¾ cup wheat berries for 24 hours)
1 cup raisins
4 tbsp shredded coconut
2 tbsp apple juice or water

Blend nuts briefly. Then add the wheat berries, raisins and coconut. Blend till smooth adding additional apple juice if necessary. Put in fridge and when cold, mould into balls and roll in coconut.

Almond and Sesame Loaf

1½ cups ground sesame seeds
1 cup finely grated carrots
1 cup finely chopped celery
½ cup finely minced red or yellow bell pepper
¼ cup finely minced red or green onion
½ cup ground almonds
1 tbsp flaxseed meal
½ tsp paprika
Pinch salt
Water

Put everything in a bowl, then slowly mix in water to make a stiff dough. Mould into oiled loaf tin and leave covered for an hour, then turn out onto a plate.

Nut and Seed Bread

1 cup hulled sunflower seeds
1 cup almonds
1 cup pumpkin seeds
1 large carrot
½ red pepper
½ cup sweet red onion
1 peeled garlic clove
¼ cup fresh parsley

Soak seeds and almonds overnight. Put the seeds, almonds, garlic and carrot in the blender. Blend well and then add the minced parsley and finely chopped red pepper and onion. Blend all together.

Then mix the following in a blender:

2 medium tomatoes
1 tsp salt
1 tbsp dried basil
1 tbsp dried oregano

Stir half of this into the bread mixture, then form into a loaf, cover and set aside for 3 hours. When ready to eat pour the rest of the tomato mix onto the loaf.

Walnut Pate

3 cups soaked walnuts
⅛ - ¼ cup soy sauce
Pinch of salt
Pinch of ground cumin
Small bunch fresh cilantro leaves
2 spring onions
2 carrots
2 celery stalks

Blend until smooth.

Pasta Squash

1 small butternut squash
1 tbsp olive oil
Pinch salt
2 tbsp shredded coconut
½ tsp curry powder
¼ tsp chili powder
Small lump fresh ginger finely chopped
1 tbsp water
1 tsp agave nectar

Deseed and skin squash. Then use a spiralizer or peeler to make noodles. Stir in olive oil and sprinkle on salt. Separately mix coconut, curry, chili, ginger and water and stir together.

Mix coconut and agave with the squash and then stir in coconut mix.

Joan's Mix

3 cups walnuts, soaked for 18 hours
3 cups chopped carrots
1 small chopped onion
1 cup chopped celery
½ cup fresh parsley
½ cup fresh basil
2 peeled garlic cloves
Juice from ½ lemon
Pinch salt

Blend walnuts and carrots until smooth.

Separately blend garlic, onion, celery, salt, herbs and lemon juice in a food processor until fairly smooth.

Mix the two lots together with a spoon.

5. SALADS

Long gone are the days where a salad consists of just lettuce, tomato and cucumber. With the vast variety of fresh produce available in our supermarkets and at specialist shops, salads can be packed full of as much flavour and goodness as you can pile on.

A simple handful of leaves and herbs is so lovely to look at that making a salad is more about getting the balance between ingredients right than thinking too hard about the actual ingredients.

Most salads are probably eaten as a side dish to a main meal but really there is no reason stopping you making them bigger and having a nice salad on its own.

Nasturtium or borage flowers make a great looking salad even better and help with that inspiration that always should go with all food preparation. Food should look attractive as well as taste good.

Celery Sultana and Nut Salad

2 chopped celery stalks
½ avocado peeled and stoned
2 tsp olive oil
Handful soaked cashew nuts
Handful sultanas

Mash the avocado and olive oil with a fork. Add the rest of the ingredients, mix well and serve.

Carrot Salad

3 carrots
½ cup raisins
1 apple, peeled and cored
1 celery stalk

Grate the peeled carrots and apple, add the finely chopped celery. Mix all ingredients in a bowl.

Dressing:

1 apple, peeled and cored
2 cups grated peeled carrot
½ cup almonds
1 tbsp apple juice

Blend until creamy and pour over salad.

Endive and Onion Salad

6 heads of endive leaves, separated
1 red onion, sliced
6oz Roquefort or Dolcelatte cheese, flaked
½ cup halved walnuts
1 tsp red wine vinegar
1 tsp walnut oil
2 tsp grape seed oil
Pinch salt and pepper
1 tsp raw honey

First make the dressing — the vinegar, oils, salt, pepper, honey and nuts by stirring them all together in a bowl.

Mix the salad together and then pour on the dressing, stir in a bowl and serve.

Nice Little Salad

Start with green leaf lettuce and/or other greens like spinach, kale, or endive and tear into small, bite-sized pieces. Fill the bowl half full of greens, then add layers of the following vegetables:

Small broccoli florets, small cauliflower florets, finely diced celery, top with grated carrots, finely diced red or yellow peppers, finely chopped sweet onion or scallions, peeled and chopped avocado.

Sea Salad

1½ cups almonds,soaked for 6 hours
3 shredded medium carrots
1 chopped red bell pepper
1 chopped green onion
2 chopped celery stalks

Put everything in blender adding a little water if necessary as you blend. Pour contents into a bowl and add the following:

½ tsp ground cumin
½ tsp dried basil
1 tsp kelp powder or 1 tbsp dried mixed
    seaweed
Pinch salt

Mix everything together then put in the fridge for 45 minutes before eating.

Avocado and Cucumber Salad

2 large peeled cucumbers chopped into ½
   inch cubes
1 small shallot sliced into very thin strips
Pinch salt
Juice from small lemon
2 cloves finely chopped peeled garlic
1 avocado chopped into ½ inch cubes

Mix all together and serve in a bowl.

Fruit and Almond Salad

1 cored and chopped apple
¼ cup almonds
Juice from ½ lemon
Water

Put everything in a blender. Begin slowly adding enough water until the mixture is smooth, fluffy, and looks like whipped cream.

Pour this sauce over a bowl of:

1 sliced banana
20 grapes — red or white

Sweet Potato Salad

Peel and finely shred 2 or 3 raw sweet potatoes.

Add 4 chopped dates and then stir in:

⅓ cup finely chopped apples
2 tbsp coarsely chopped walnuts
1 tsp orange zest
¼ cup fresh orange juice

Put in a bowl and enjoy.

Tomato and Basil Salad

3-4 medium tomatoes cut into ½ inch pieces
2 garlic cloves peeled and chopped very small
½ cup fresh basil leaves finely chopped
2 tbsp olive oil
½ tsp salt

Put all together and leave in fridge for 45 minutes before eating.

Pecan, Pear and Apple Salad

2 red delicious apples
1 yellow delicious apple
1 pear
3 celery sticks
¼ cup chopped dates
½ cup chopped pecans
1 orange
1 lemon

Chop celery finely, then peel and chop apples and pears into small pieces. Juice lemon and orange and pour over the mix to keep them from turning brown. Stir to coat all fruit, and allow to stand for 10 minutes. Then drain, saving the juice. Meanwhile chop pecans and dates and then add half of the chopped pecans along with the dates and celery to the drained fruit.

Put the rest of the pecans in a blender, along with the juice drained from the fruit then add this sauce to the salad and stir to blend all the flavor

Apple Salad

4 juicy apples
¼ cup raisins
¼ cup sliced almonds
¼ cup oatmeal
Pinch cinnamon, allspice and nutmeg
⅛ cup maple syrup

Core and cut up apples and place in mixing bowl. Add remaining ingredients except for maple syrup and stir thoroughly.

Drizzle maple syrup over apples and other ingredients just prior to serving and mix well.

6. VEGETABLES

Eating vegetables raw, if they are not already part of your meals or snacks at present, may seem quite a strange addition to your diet, but it really doesn't have to feel like rabbit food.

It's easy to make things that little bit more interesting than nibbling through whole carrots and celery sticks. Although many vegetables (peeled and chopped carrots, sprigs of broccoli and cauliflower, celery, etc.) are a great snack on their own for some people, it can feel like a real effort for others.

There is also the option of sauces and dressings to make the vegetable of choice that bit more interesting and grating and very fine chopping are actions that work very well.

A large plate of raw fibrous vegetables such as green beans, broccoli, cauliflower, etc. may seem too much of a challenge, so lightly steaming just to gently soften them is better than cooking fully and definitely better than not having them at all. Not totally raw, but near enough to start with.

Lettuce Taco Wrap

2 avocados peeled and stoned
1 red onion
¼ cup fresh lemon juice
1 oz fresh parsley, chopped
½ tsp cumin
2 chopped garlic cloves
1 cup chopped sun-dried tomatoes,
   soaked for 2 hours
3 chopped jalapenos
1½ tsp sea salt
Leaf lettuce

Slice the avocados and slosh lemon juice over them. Chop the onion in food processor first and then add the rest and blend until smooth. Place a dollop into a lettuce leaf and wrap the leaf around the mixture.

Salsa

6 chopped medium tomatoes
½ cup chopped onion
1 small pepper chopped
4 celery stalks, minced

Mix them all together and allow to stand
for one hour.

Then add:

½ cup olive oil
A few chopped nuts or seeds
2 minced garlic cloves
½ cup basil leaves

Stir and put in fridge for 45 minute then
pour on the juice from a lemon and eat.

Spaghetti

2 large zucchini peeled and coarsely grated

Put the following in a blender:

2 cloves peeled garlic
2 ripe medium tomatoes
½ cup sun dried tomatoes
2 tbsp extra virgin olive oil
¼ cup fresh basil
¼ cup fresh oregano
1 tsp salt

Blend well and pour over the zucchini.

Avocado and Cucumber Spread

1 mashed avocado
½ grated cucumber
Juice of ½ lemon
Pinch unrefined sea salt
Pinch black pepper

Mix all together and mash with a fork and spread on bread or crackers.

Beetroot and Carrot Bowl

Finely grate two medium carrots and one smallish beetroot. That's it!

Optional extras:

Grate small piece of ginger onto the mix.
Squeeze an orange over.
Drizzle with oil.

Combine with any sauce, dressing or dip.

Sweet Potato Mousse

2½ cups peeled and chopped sweet potatoes
10 stoned dates
1 tsp vanilla extract
1 tsp ground cinnamon
1½ cups Water
1 tbsp coconut oil
½ tsp Psyllium
Pinch salt
½ cup chopped pecans

Blend dates, vanilla extract, cinnamon, salt, coconut oil, and water. Now put in the sweet potatoes and blend until smooth. Add Psyllium (one to check out) and blend well. Leave for a few minutes. Blend again until smooth and sprinkle with the pecans.

Coleslaw

½ very thinly sliced white cabbage
3 roughly grated medium carrots
Dessing of choice, like a mayonnaise
Pinch salt
Pinch pepper

Put everything in a large bowl and mix together.

Herby Tomatoes

Slice up tomatoes.

Chop up herb leaves such as basil, fennel, cilantro, mint, parsley and sprinkle on with a drizzle of olive oil.

Olives and Sun-dried Tomatoes

Olives and sun-dried tomatoes are so tempting and are pretty much raw. Depending on how fussy you want to be, they can be a great snack or part of almost any meal. Check the label or ask at the deli counter about production.

7. SAUCES, DIPS AND DRESSINGS

Sauces, dips and dressings can really lift recipes and make even an ordinary lettuce leaf very interesting and exciting. There are lots of different styles of dips but they all need to be eaten within a couple of days to be at their best. They should not be allowed to dry out at all.

Try them with vegetables as well as salads and start to incorporate them in the mixture not only as a poured on item but fully stirred in. Here is a selection of some of the best.

Guacamole

1 ripe chopped avocado
1 clove of crushed peeled garlic
1 tsp fresh lime juice
1 heaped tsp of onion, finely chopped
Pinch salt
Ground cayenne

Place all the ingredients in a bowl and mash with a fork or, for a smooth creamy texture, use a hand blender for a couple of seconds. Sprinkle with cayenne.

Houmus

9oz sprouted chick peas
2 tbsp tahini
2 tbsp extra virgin olive oil
1 tbsp lemon juice
1 tbsp tamari
2 cloves peeled garlic
2 tbsp water

Place all the ingredients into a blender and blend until smooth.

Carrot Dip

4 medium sized carrots peeled and chopped
½ large chopped onion
2 tbsp lemon juice
2 tbsp extra virgin olive oil
4 tbsp tahini
2 tbsp water

Blend everything until smooth.
Finely chopped dill can be added for taste.

Cranberry Sauce

8oz fresh cranberries
1 peeled orange
1 peeled and cored apple
4oz fresh stoned dates
Water

Put cranberries, orange, apple and dates in a blender till smooth - add water if needed.

Pesto

60 fresh basil leaves
Juice from ½ lemon
4 cloves peeled garlic
1 cup pine nuts
½ tsp salt
½ cup olive oil

Clean and wash basil, crush garlic very fine then add all ingredients and blend.

Pea with Mint

Defrost a handful of frozen peas. Blend them to a thick sauce, then add a handful of chopped mint and blend briefly again.

Chutney

3 apples peeled, cored and chopped
1 onion peeled and chopped
1½ tsp ground coriander
⅓ cup raisins, soaked for 20 mins and
    strained
½ cup cider vinegar

Blend briefly, put in a jar and keep in fridge.

Garlic Olive Oil

1 pint extra virgin olive oil
3 large garlic cloves, peeled and crushed

Put garlic in the olive oil bottle. Use on salads.

Tomato Delight

1 large avocado cut into cubes
1 chopped medium tomato
1 small chopped peeled cucumber
Juice from ½ lemon or lime
½ tsp salt
1 tsp olive oil

Blend all and serve in small bowls.

Tahini Dressing

4oz of raw tahini
Juice from ½ lemon
1 peeled garlic clove
¼ tsp cayenne pepper
½ tsp soy sauce

Blend all ingredients with enough water to make a nice dressing.

Apple Sauce

3 apples
1 banana
4 soft dates
¼ cup water

Blend all ingredients with a little bit of grated nutmeg.

Sunflower and Lemon Dressing

2½ cups water
1½ cups raw hulled sunflower seeds
1 tsp salt
2 tsp paprika
2 tsp onion powder (or flakes)
Juice from 2 lemons
1 finely chopped clove peeled garlic

Blend until very creamy.

Poppy Seed Salad Topping

4 tbsp lemon juice
4 tbsp orange juice
½ cup soaked almonds
2 tbsp green onion
½ tsp ground paprika
2 tbsp poppy seeds

Soak almonds overnight. Put everything in the blender except the poppy seeds. Sprinkle on the poppy seeds when serving.

Fine Salad Dressing

½ peeled avocado
1 celery stalk
1 tomato
¼ cup fresh chopped chives
¼ cup fresh chopped parsley
½ cup coarsely chopped onion
1 cup water
¼ cup cider vinegar
Pinch salt

Combine all ingredients in blender until smooth.

Fine Garlic Salad Dressing

1 cup extra virgin olive oil
¼ cup apple cider vinegar
¼ cup soy sauce
¼ cup honey
Chopped ginger to taste
2 chopped peeled garlic cloves

Put all ingredients in blender for one
minute and put in a jar for storage.

Simple Salad Dressing

4 tbsp hemp seed oil
2 tbsp lemon juice
1½ tbsp raw soy sauce
1 tbsp raw honey

Whisk everything together and use on
any salad.

8. NUTS AND SEEDS

Nuts and seeds are a great source of protein, vitamins, minerals and essential amino acids, so becoming an important part of your new diet.

Do stay away from salted nuts however as they are usually over processed. It's easy to sprinkle salt on to your own. Nuts and seeds are best eaten before they are eight months old. A lot of produce on the shelves can be older than this so check if you can.

Man has been chewing and eating and enjoying a huge range of these foods for tens of thousands of years and although our ancestor's teeth were undoubtedly stronger than ours we can benefit from them by using our blenders and grinders and also the simple pestle and mortar.

It's a good idea to soak nuts in purified water for up to twenty-four hours as this gets the germination process going which makes them even more nutritious.

Here is a list of the most popular and easiest to find nuts:

Almonds
Brazils
Cashews
Coconuts
Filberts
Hazelnuts
Macadamia
Peanuts
Pecans
Pine Kernels
Pistacchio
Walnuts

They can all be eaten on their own or used in many recipes, some of which are here.

Here is a list of the most popular and edible seeds:

Anise
Caraway
Coriander
Fennel
Fenugreek
Flax
Hemp
Marrow
Poppy
Pumpkin
Sesame
Sunflower

These can be eaten on their own during the day at anytime or mixed with or sprinkled on most foods and salads.

Fine Almond Spread

2 tbsp ground almonds
1 tsp honey
2 tbsp yeast
Pinch salt
2 tbsp water

Mix in small bowl and serve.

Macadamia Salad Dressing

⅓ cup pure macadamia oil
2 tbsp vinegar
2 cloves fresh peeled garlic
1 tsp fresh chopped parsley

Crush garlic and put ingredients in a jar and shake well.

Almond Milk

2 cup almonds, soaked for 6 – 8 hours
6 cups water
3 stoned dates

Combine almonds and water in a blender until smooth.

Strain the blended mixture through two layers of cheese cloth. Add the dates and reblend.

Keep in fridge, otherwise this mixture will ferment in a warm place in a few hours.

Macadamia and Peach Pie

1 cup macadamias, halves and pieces
1 cup fresh ricotta cheese
1 cup fromage frais
2 tbsp agave nectar
3 cups sliced fresh peaches
1 tsp water

Using electric beaters, whip together the ricotta, fromage frais, water and agave nectar until thick and fluffy. Put a layer of the peaches on a plate, top with some of the ricotta mixture and sprinkle with the macadamias. Repeat making many layers. Sprinkle the top with the rest of the chopped macadamias.

Nut Paté

1 cup cashew nuts
½ cup almonds
½ peeled and chopped onion
1 tbsp soya sauce
½ red bell pepper
12 fresh basil leaves
¼ cup water
1 cup dried banana slices
1 tbsp raw agave nectar
Pinch ground cinnamon
½ cup chopped walnuts
Pinch salt
Pinch nutmeg

Soak the nuts in water for one hour, until the cashews become soft and the almonds plump up. Once the nuts are soaked put into blender with all the rest of the ingredients. When adding the onion, also pour in about 1 tablespoon of the soya sauce for flavor. Blend slowly so that the mixture does get too sloppy.

Now add the banana and agave nectar with a pinch of salt and cinnamon.

Put the walnuts, salt, cinnamon, and nutmeg in now and carry on till you get a doughy consistency to the mix. Mould in your hands into small cookies.

Raw Almonds

If you've never tried snacking on raw almonds, you're really missing out. In fact, raw almonds are some of the healthiest, most nutritionally-dense, energy-packed fitness superfoods available. Best of all, almonds have more dietary fibre and more calcium than any other nut — great for anyone looking to lose weight.

Walnut Roll

1½ cups raw walnuts
1½ tsp ground cumin
¾ tsp ground coriander
2 tsp soy sauce
Pinch cayenne

Grind the walnuts in food processor to fine crumb texture and stir in everything else and roll it up in a large lettuce leaf.

Pear and Walnut Salad

3 ripe pears
1 tbsp lemon juice
3 tbsps walnut, hazelnut or olive oil
¼ cup chopped walnuts
Fresh ground black pepper

Peel the pears. Slice them in half, take out the core then slice each pear half into four. Put the pear slices in a bowl, add the lemon juice and oil to the pears and stir once. Divide up the salad onto plates and top with walnuts and a little ground black pepper.

Sunflower Seed Cream

1 cup sunflower seeds
1 cup of water
4 tsp lemon juice
1 pressed peeled garlic clove
¾ tsp onion powder
Pinch salt

Blend all ingredients together until smooth.

Sunflower Mix

2 cups sunflower seeds soaked for 20
    minutes
¾ cup fresh dill
2 tbsps fresh lemon juice
2 cloves peeled garlic
½ cup water

Put all in blender till smooth and serve with finely sliced carrots.

Nut Butter

1½ cups nuts: Almonds, walnuts,
    cashews, peanuts or pecans
Flax oil, as needed
Pinch salt

Powder nuts or seeds in a grinder. The powder should be as fine as you can get it although a few larger crumbs are alright.

Put in blender and while it is going, add oil until it looks smooth. It will solidify a bit once it's stored so better softer than harder. Add a pinch of salt and put in a jar to keep in the fridge. It will need stirring before use.

Trail Mix

When you are out walking or cycling and enjoying the great outdoors trail mix is well known for keeping you going. Rather than buy a readymade mix the best option is to make up your own. Here is a list of some key ingredients that most mixes contain. Pick and choose to find the combination that you like best to keep in your pocket:

Almonds
Brazil nuts
Cashews
Dates
Figs
Dried apple
Dried apricots
Dried banana chips
Filberts
Peanuts
Pistachio nuts
Pumpkin seeds
Raisins and currants
Sesame seeds
Shredded coconut
Sunflower seeds
Walnuts
Whole oats

Sprouting Seeds

Sprouting seeds takes a good few hours, which sometimes puts people off trying themselves as it isn't instant. But they're really low maintenance and once you work out that you can start some soaking before you go to bed and they will be ready when you wake up, you'll soon realise they're effortless. It's just a case of getting into the habit of soaking and sprouting.

Sprouts are one of the most complete and nutritional of all foods. Sprouts are rich in vitamins, minerals, proteins, and enzymes. Their nutritional value has been known by the Chinese for thousands of years.

As an example, a sprouted Mung bean has the carbohydrate content of a melon, vitamin A of a lemon, thiamin of an avocado, riboflavin of a dry apple, niacin of a banana, and ascorbic acid of a loganberry.

To make a sprouting container is easy. Just use an old, clean wide mouthed jar or container with a cover that lets some air in. Or buy one online.

Seeds are readily available and the most common types are:

Alfalfa
Chickpea
Cress and curly cress
Mung beans

All you need do is rinse the seeds and put in the container. Keep them somewhere dark and warm and remember to rinse them every day in cold water. Once sprouted rinse them off and keep in the fridge. They only keep for a few days.

9. DESSERTS

Those of us with a sweet tooth always are on the lookout for something to finish a meal or have as an item to sustain us through long foodless times.

Throughout history we have tried to find the fulfilment and pleasure of a good sweet thing. Eating a piece of fruit is an obvious answer, but here are some ideas for the kind of satisfactory sensation that makes the hunt worthwhile.

.

Mango Delight

2 mangos
½ peeled and deseeded lime
2oz shredded coconut
2oz chopped pecans

Peel mangos and remove the stones. Add lime and blend well.

Pour into bowls and top with the coconut and pecans.

Evening Thing

2 peeled sliced bananas
1 skinned stoned peeled mango
10 strawberries
2 stoned dates

Put everything in a food processor and blend — serve in bowls.

Banana Ice Cream

Peel two ripe bananas and put them in your freezer for 4 hours. Then take them out and blend them with one or two peeled and stoned frozen mangos. Eat straightaway.

Raisin and Fig Dessert

2 cups sprouted wheat and rye mixed
1½ cups black figs, soaked overnight
1½ cups raisins, soaked in fig water for
    1 hour.

Blend all together until smooth.

Avocado Choc Pudding

3 ripe avocados, peeled and stoned
½ cup almond milk
⅓ cup maple syrup
⅓ cup dark cocoa powder
¼ tsp ground cinnamon
Put everything in a blender or food processor until creamy.

Fruit Salad

This is a quick and easy snack or dessert that can be made in bulk to last a couple of days to be dipped into when required. Just put in whatever fruits you have available.

Nutty Maple Pie

2 cups pecan nuts
4 tbsp organic maple syrup
1 tsp pure vanilla extract

Blend nuts until a fine texture is reached.
Then add maple syrup and vanilla, a bit
at a time, until nuts coalesce then mould
into a pie plate.

Fill with any chopped fruit.

Banana Thrill

½ cup cocoa powder
¼ cup fresh stoned dates
3 chilled bananas
1 cup hazelnuts

Blend until smooth.

Honey and Honeycomb

The oldest natural dessert in the world — and still as good as ever. Some honey is heat treated when it is being prepared but any locally produced honey is normally extracted from the comb on a warm summer's day so does not need heat to extract it and so is raw.

Honeycomb is just the best and can be added to most desserts to make a fabulous extravagant taste. Eaten with a spoon on its own is a favorite!

Agave Syrup

Agave syrup or nectar is sometimes heated during extraction so check the label.

Nice Fudge

1 cup rolled oats
¾ cup carob powder
¼ cup ground sesame seed
¼ cup ground sunflower seeds
½ cup almond butter
5 stoned dates soaked for an hour
¾ to 1 cup chopped walnuts

Place everything in blender with S blade.
Pour into flat pan and refrigerate before
serving.

Brownies

1 cup ground pecans
1 cup dried dates
¼ cup cocao powder
1 tsp agave nectar

For the topping:

1 tbsp coconut oil or coconut butter
1 tbsp agave
½ tbsp cocao powder

Blend brownie ingredients and press into shallow dish then blend all the topping together and spread onto brownies and keep in fridge.

Pecan Cookies

1 cup raw pecan butter
20 pitted medjool dates
¾ cup shredded dried coconut
Pinch salt
1 tbsp cacao nibs

Blend dates until smooth. Then blend in
pecan butter, coconut and salt. Stir in
the cacao nibs then shape into cookies
and keep in fridge.

Untreated Milk

Although not strictly a dessert this is a raw foodstuff that's worth checking out. There are dairies that specialise in producing raw untreated milk fresh from the cow and who have struggled against regulations to make all milk heat treated. There are health considerations for you to think about but raw milk can be good on its own or flavored.

Cheese and yoghurt from raw milk can be included in your diet and it's very easy to make your own cottage cheese if you feel adventurous. Different areas have different regulations.

Notes, Ideas and Recipes

Notes, Ideas and Recipes

Notes, Ideas and Recipes

Notes, Ideas and Recipes

Notes, Ideas and Recipes

Notes, Ideas and Recipes

Notes, Ideas and Recipes

INDEX